DISABLED PERSONS (SERVICES, CONSULTATION AND REPRESENTATION) ACT 1986

THIRTEENTH REPORT ON THE DEVELOPMENT OF SERVICES FOR PEOPLE WITH A MENTAL ILLNESS IN ENGLAND pursuant to Section 11 of the Disabled Persons (Services, Consultation and Representation) Act 1986 as amended.

This is the Thirteenth report to be laid pursuant to Section 11 of the Disabled Persons (Services, Consultation and Representation) Act 1986, as amended which requires the Secretary of State for Health to provide:

- such information as he considers appropriate with respect to the development of health and social services in the community for persons suffering from mental illness who are not resident in hospital;

- information with respect to persons receiving in-patient treatment for mental illness in health service hospitals; and

- such other information as he considers appropriate.

This report is in two parts:

Section A: describes the broad development of mental health services since the Victorian age; and

Section B: describes the background to the current policy and the developments in mental health services that have taken place since the Twelfth report.

SECTION A: THE BROAD DEVELOPMENT OF MENTAL HEALTH SERVICES SINCE THE VICTORIAN AGE.

1. The Victorians who created enormous mental asylums were undoubtedly well intentioned. Sadly, the new "hospitals" quickly became overcrowded and people continued to be held, in largely unchanged conditions, throughout the first half of the twentieth century.

2. When the NHS inherited these institutions, life in them was still poor. In the post-war years new, more effective, medication became available and the number of people in hospital started to decline. A Royal Commission led to the Mental Health Act of 1959, and to people receiving care outside of the traditional hospital setting.

3. A different pattern of mental health care grew slowly from the 1960s onwards. Many places introduced day hospitals, and from the 1970s acute wards in district general hospitals offered an alternative to institutionalisation.

4. The 1980s saw the start of community mental health teams. Increasingly, non governmental organisations, such as MIND and the National Schizophrenia Fellowship (now Rethink), developed initiatives where people in the community could socialise, get information and help and develop a sense of self-worth and empowerment.

5. By the late 1980s, the large hospitals had started to close and those that remained were a fraction of their former size. The policies set out in a Government White Paper in 1975 *Better Services for the Mentally Ill* had, however, failed to materialise in most places.

6. In a few areas innovative new services were introduced but overall, progress was patchy and poor. Services were not meeting needs comprehensively and those that tried to do so often relied heavily on the commitment of a few pioneering individuals.

7. In the NHS, mental health remained a poor relation among services. Joint planning between health and local authorities was often ineffective and the views of those who used services were rarely sought – and almost never heeded.

8. The 1990s were not easy times for mental health. Increasingly, staff had to tackle not just mental illness, but drugs, alcohol and violence. Many became frustrated and concerned by the limitations on what they could provide.

9. With the old asylums closing and their resources not always reinvested in mental health care, the community too often became a bleak and neglected environment for people with mental health problems.

10. Hospital beds came under pressure and as the number fell patients were often sent to anywhere that could take them. Shabby, depressing wards – that would never have been tolerated in medicine or surgery – were still common place in mental hospitals. Staff morale was low, and the stigma of being ill remained high.

11. Several important reports and enquiries in the 1990s found that there were still many defects in mental health services. These included poor communication between the responsible agencies, especially health and social services, and the inadequate use of care plans. One report described the 'chaos of community care' – which echoed the experience of many.

DISABLED PERSONS (SERVICES, CONSULTATION AND REPRESENTATION) ACT 1986

Development of Services for People with a Mental Illness in England

Thirteenth report prepared pursuant to Section 11 of the Disabled Persons (Services, Consultation and Representation) Act 1986 as amended

Pursuant to c.33 1986 Section 11

Ordered by the House of Commons *to be printed 15 September 2003*

LONDON: The Stationery Office
£6.50

HC 1036

SECTION B: THE BACKGROUND TO THE CURRENT POLICY AND THE DEVELOPMENTS IN MENTAL HEALTH SERVICES THAT HAVE TAKEN PLACE SINCE THE TWELFTH REPORT.

NEW POLICIES FOR THE MILLENNIUM

12. The Government has responded by making mental health one of the top three health priorities – alongside coronary heart disease and cancer. The main planks of its new policies which together, state a clear and comprehensive plan for mental health services are:

- the white paper *Modernising Mental Health Services*
- *The National Service Framework for Mental Health*
- the chapter on mental health in the NHS Plan
- a review of the *Mental Health Act 1983*.

13. The new policies were heralded in the 1998 White Paper, Modernising Mental Health Services, which proposes local mental health and social services that are:

Modernising Mental Health Services

- **safe** – to protect patients and the public and provide effective care for those with mental illness at the time they need it;

- **sound** – ensuring that patients and service users have access to the full range of services which they need; and

- **supportive** – working with patients and service users, their families and carers, to build healthier communities.

14. The White Paper set ten guiding principles. People with mental health problems can expect services that will:

- involve users and their carers in the planning and delivery of care;

- deliver high quality treatment and care, which is known to be effective and acceptable;

- be well suited to those who use them and be non-discriminatory;

- be accessible, so that help can be obtained when and where it is needed;

- promote their safety and that of their carers, staff and the wider public;

- offer choices which promote independence;

- be well co-ordinated between all staff and agencies;

- deliver continuity of care for as long as it is needed;

- empower and support staff;

- be properly accountable to the public, users and carers; and

- reduce suicides.

The National Service Framework

15. The *National Service Framework for Mental Health* (NSF) was published in September 1999. It set out a ten-year programme to put in place new high standards of care, which people can be entitled to expect in every part of the country.

16. The NSF fleshed out the policies in Modernising Mental Health Services, by defining models of care and treatment. It also sets milestones and targets against which progress, within time-scales, is being measured.

17. The aims of the National Service Framework standards are:

- *Mental health promotion* – to ensure health and social services promote mental health and reduce the discrimination and social exclusion associated with mental health problems;

- *Primary care and access to services* – to deliver better primary mental health care, and to ensure consistent advice and help for people with mental health needs, including primary care services for individuals with severe mental illness;

- *Effective services for people with severe mental illness* – to ensure that each person with severe mental illness receives the range of mental health services they need; that crises are anticipated or prevented where possible; to ensure prompt and effective help if a crisis does occur, and timely access to an appropriate and safe mental health place or hospital bed, as close to home as possible;

- *Caring about carers* – to ensure health and social services assess the needs of carers who provide regular and substantial care for those with severe mental illness, and provide care to meet their needs; and

- *Preventing suicide* – to ensure that health and social services play their full part in reducing the suicide rate by at least one fifth by 2010.

The NHS Plan

18. This was published in July 2000 as a programme of radical reform of the NHS. The *NHS Plan* makes a number of pledges for mental health including assertive outreach, home treatment and early intervention services for all who need them, more help for people held inappropriately in high secure hospitals or prison, new services for women, and more support for carers.

The NHS Plan will create, by 2004:

- 1000 new graduate mental health staff to work in primary care;

- an extra 500 community mental health team workers;

- 50 early intervention teams to provide treatment and support to young people with psychosis and their families;

- 335 crisis resolution teams;

- an increase to 220 assertive outreach teams;

- women only day services;

- 700 extra staff to work with carers;

- more suitable accommodation for up to 400 people currently in high secure hospital;

- better services for prisoners with mental illness; and

- a care plan and keyworker for every prisoner leaving prison with serious mental illness.

19. Whenever possible, people with mental health problems should be treated without the use of any compulsion. When this is not possible, a modern mental health service must be supported by legislation that reflects new patterns of care and treatment, respects civil liberties, and promotes effective recovery.

Reform of the Mental Health Act

20. Current mental health law was conceived in the 1950s, with some revision in 1983. The Draft Mental Health Bill and Consultation Document (published for consultation on 25 June 2002), put forward proposals, for a modern legal framework and introduces new safeguards for service users and more focus on their individual needs. Nearly 2000 responses have been received to the consultation exercise, which are currently being considered. The Government intends to introduce legislation as soon as Parliamentary time allows.

Proposed changes in mental health law include:

- the introduction of a new tribunal system, to authorise any use of long term compulsion only on the basis of assessed needs and individual care and treatment plans;

- the possibility of compulsory orders being based in the community, rather than just in hospital; and

- new specialist independent advocacy services available to anyone who is being treated under the Act.

21. The system for the use of compulsory powers will also be simplified. This will make it clearer when compulsory treatment may be appropriate, due to the risk of self-harm or due to the substantial risk of significant harm to others.

WHAT MAKES THESE POLICIES SO DIFFERENT?

- The people who use mental health services will be involved, as equal partners and at every level, to ensure the new services make sense;

- new policies address the whole range of needs of people with mental health difficulties – from care plans to citizenship;

- substantial new money is being provided;

- clear targets have been set, and a timetable for achieving them over the next ten years;

- new national and local groups have been made responsible for seeing that this happens.

Help at the onset of illness   22. Some serious mental health difficulties, such as schizophrenia, usually first occur during teenage years or the early twenties. Often young people will be unwell for six months or more before they get any help. To remedy this situation, early intervention teams will be able to provide the intensive support and help that every young person who develops a first episode of psychosis needs. These teams operate in ways that young people can relate to, providing help and advice on managing symptoms, and will base their care on the belief that engagement, rather than compulsion, is the key to success.

Help in a crisis   23. At the moment, the only option for most people needing urgent mental health care is admission to hospital. Often this results in too long a period away from home, work and social networks, and can mean that all of these are damaged or lost. In some areas, special crisis resolution teams make an urgent visit to anyone who is thought to need to go into hospital. Often, the crisis can then be resolved, and by providing intensive treatment at home, a great many hospital admissions can be avoided. This type of service is one that many people prefer.

Help for frequent users   24. A small number of people use a lot of mental health services. They are frequently admitted to hospital, often compulsorily, but sometimes lose touch with services soon after discharge. Often they suffer from a dual diagnosis of substance misuse and serious mental illness. A small proportion also have a history of offending. For this group, assertive outreach teams providing intensive support at home can keep in touch with them, reduce the amount of time they spend in hospital, and help them enjoy a better quality of life.

Community teams   25. Community mental health teams (CMHTs) will continue to have an important role to play in supporting service users and families in community settings. They should provide the core around which modern mental health services are developed. Their responsibilities may change over time but, working with primary care, they will be the main pathway for referrals to the more specialist teams. CMHTs, in some places known as primary care liaison teams, will also continue to care for the majority of people with moderate to severe mental illness in the community.

Better help in hospital   26. Hospitals will also continue to play an important part in mental health care. An effective support system must get the balance right, between better community-based care and high quality, therapeutic inpatient care in good accommodation.

The NHS has been set three national objectives that are:

- to ensure good standards of dignity and privacy for hospital patients;

- to achieve the Patient's Charter standards for segregated washing and toilet facilities;

- safe hospital facilities for patients who are mentally unwell.

WHAT IT MEANS

…for society   27. Mental illness can be experienced at any time. One in four people will do so during the course of their lives. The Government aims to reduce that figure by improving the mental well being of the general population, especially people who are most vulnerable to mental ill health. Another aim is to reduce the stigma and discrimination that faces those who fall ill, and so work against social exclusion or marginalization.

A campaign called "mind out for mental health" has been launched to challenge discrimination by raising awareness of mental health, starting with employers, the media and young people.

28. One of the biggest problems people face when they experience mental health difficulties is keeping a job – or getting (back to) work afterwards. Research undertaken for the Government has shown a poor understanding among employers about mental health issues. The *mind out for mental health* campaign includes a programme – *working minds* – to challenge discrimination in the workplace against people with mental health problems.

The NHS will set an example – health and social services have been asked to promote the employment of people with mental health problems in the services they provide.

29. Greater opportunities will also be sought for people with mental health problems to access suitable housing, education, welfare benefits and other services, to help empower them to participate in society.

Local services have been asked to develop mental health promotion strategies, based on local needs, including action in specific settings which could include schools, the workplace and prisons. The plans must also include action at a local level to reduce discrimination.

30. Health and social services should: **NSF standard one**

- promote mental health for all, working with individuals and communities;

- combat discrimination against individuals and groups with mental health problems, and promote their social inclusion.

Action taken since the last report includes

31. In August 2001, the Department of Health published *Making It Happen: A guide to delivering mental health promotion*. The document was developed in extensive consultation with a wide variety of stakeholders from the field and is intended to be helpful rather than prescriptive. It is designed to provide practical advice to help health and social services promote mental health by:

- defining mental health and mental health promotion;

- making the case for investing in mental health promotion;

- showing how mental health promotion fits in with other policy initiatives;

- providing a framework for developing local strategies;

- describing the types of evidence and their strengths and weaknesses;

- giving examples of effective intervention;

- describing how to apply the evidence;

- giving information on evaluation.

32. The Department of Health's *mind out for mental health* campaign, launched in March 2001, is a sustained programme of activity which aims to tackle the stigma and discrimination faced by people with mental health problems. The campaign supports the implementation of Standard One of the National Service Framework for Mental Health. *mind out for mental health works* alongside partners in the voluntary sector, the media and business to change attitudes and behaviour surrounding mental health. The campaign targets three particular groups: employers, young people and the media as well as the public at large. In June, the campaign website was launched - www.mindout.net.

33. 'Working Minds' is the employer programme of *mind out for mental health*. This part of the campaign works in partnership with employers to help improve workplace policy and practice on mental health. On 19 June 2001 two elements of the employer programme were launched:

- **research** carried out for by the Industrial Society entitled 'Attitudes on mental health with proposals for change'. This revealed that employers and employees have a lack of understanding and awareness of mental health, and that people with mental health problems face discrimination at work;

- **a toolkit** designed as a practical resource for human resource professionals. It included a strong business case detailing why mental health should be on the corporate agenda, case studies of people with a mental health problem in work, case studies of better practice employers and case studies of people who have successfully used the Disability Discrimination Act. There were also facts on mental health in the workplace, resource lists and interactive games for use by human resource professionals.

34. The Department of Health contributed £100,000 in 2001/2 to support the Department for the Environment, Food and Rural Affairs' Rural Stress Action Plan. The contribution supported local voluntary sector initiatives to alleviate stress in the rural community, exacerbated by the foot and mouth crisis.

NSF standard two

35. Any service user who contacts their primary health care team with a common mental health problem should:

- have their mental health needs identified and assessed;

- be offered effective treatments, including referral to specialist services for further assessment, treatment and care if they require it.

NSF standard three

36. Any individual with a common mental health problem should:

- be able to make contact round the clock with the local services necessary to meet their needs and receive adequate care;

- be able to use *NHS Direct*, as it develops, for first-level advice and referral on to specialist helplines or to local services.

PRIMARY CARE MENTAL HEALTH

37. Mental health problems are common and primary health care teams provide most of the help that people need. Up to 40 per cent of patients attending their GP for any reason will have a mental health problem and in 20-25 per cent of cases, a mental health problem, typically anxiety and/or depression, will be the sole reason for attending. In addition, many people with less common but more severe mental illnesses are also managed in primary care.

38. Standard two sets out how service users contacting primary health care teams should have their mental health needs identified and assessed; and be offered effective treatments, including referral to specialist services for further assessment, treatment and care if they require it.

39. Standard three sets out how those with mental health problems should be able to make contact round the clock with the local services necessary to meet their needs and receive adequate care; and be able to use *NHS Direct* for advice and onward referral.

40. Since publication of the NSF, specific targets and additional resources, have been identified in The NHS Plan (July 2000). The Plan says that by 2004, one thousand new graduate primary care mental health workers, trained in brief therapy techniques of proven effectiveness, will be appointed. The aim is to help GPs manage and treat common mental health problems in all age groups, including children.

By December 2002, guidance on graduate primary care mental health workers was in development and training was in the process of being commissioned.

41. In addition, 500 more community mental health staff will be employed by 2004 to work with GPs and primary care teams, with NHS Direct, and in each accident and emergency department. Known as 'Gateway' workers, these staff will respond to people who need immediate help, and be able to call on crisis resolution teams if necessary. Providing more help in primary care will ease the pressure on GP services helping to improve the health and well being of the population.

By December 2002, guidance on 'Gateway' workers had been published.

Action taken since the last report includes

42. In November 2001, a major conference was held for staff working in primary care and their colleagues in specialised services. Led by the Health Minister, Jacqui Smith, over 500 delegates were able to receive the latest information about work to progress the primary care mental health targets, and share views. Further information is available at www.doh.gov/fastforward.

43. For the financial year 2002/3, £2.5m central funds is being made available to support the establishment of new programmes of education and training to support the new graduate workers, and ultimately other members of primary care teams, in the delivery of effective primary care mental health. South Trent Workforce Development Confederation leads for this work, supported by the Department of Health.

44. All mental health service users on Care Programme Approach (CPA) should: **NSF standard four**

- receive care which optimises engagement, anticipates or prevents a crisis, and reduces risk

- have a copy of a written care plan which:

    - includes the action to be taken in a crisis by the service user, their carer, and their care co-ordinator;

    - advises their GP how they should respond if the service user needs additional help;

    - is regularly reviewed by their care co-ordinator;

    - be able to access services 24 hours a day, 365 days a year.

NSF standard five

45. Each service user who is assessed as requiring a period of care away from their home should have:

- timely access to an appropriate hospital bed or alternative bed or place, which is:

  - in the least restrictive environment consistent with the need to protect them and the public;

  - as close to home as possible.

- a copy of a written after care plan agreed on discharge which sets out the care and rehabilitation to be provided, identifies the care co-ordinator, and specifies the action to be taken in a crisis.

Modernising the Care Programme Approach

46. The *Care Programme Approach* (CPA) has been central to Government policy since 1991. It was seen as a crucial means to ensure that, following the closure of the old, long stay, hospitals, people with mental health problems received the care they needed, rather than lose contact with services and end up homeless or exploited.

47. CPA requires that everyone accepted for treatment or care by specialist mental health services should have their health and social care needs assessed and:

- a package of care (care plan) to meet those needs drawn up;

- a named mental health worker (care co-ordinator) to keep in close touch with them;

- a regular review of their needs and their care plan.

48. Good care planning remains the vital gateway for appropriate access to the new range of services and supports. CPA is being audited at local level, to ensure that any remaining difficulties are overcome.

Written care plans for those people on the enhanced Care Programme Approach must show plans to secure:

- *suitable employment or other occupational activity;*

- *adequate housing;*

- *appropriate entitlement to welfare benefits.*

By March 2004, this requirement will apply to everyone on CPA.

Early intervention in psychosis

49. The NHS Plan target to develop 50 Early Intervention teams by 2004 was designed to help people under the aged of thirty-five who have developed psychosis, such as schizophrenia. The teams will deliver the early and intensive support they need.

By December 2002, 22 Early Intervention teams had been set up.

By 2004, this will benefit an estimated 7,500 young people each year.

Crisis resolution

50. If the problems are so acute that people require admission to hospital, they will have the choice of earlier and more effective treatment in their own home.

51. A total of 335 crisis resolution and home treatment teams were proposed in the NHS Plan for establishment by 2004. The aim is to treat an estimated 100,000 people a year who would otherwise have to be admitted to hospital. The demand for beds will be reduced by 30% and there will generally be no admissions to distant hospitals, unless the expert care of a specialist centre is needed.

By 2004, all people in contact with specialist mental health services will be able to access crisis resolution services at any time. The Crisis Resolution Teams will deliver this. By December 2002, 86 Crisis Resolution teams had been set up.

52. The small number of people who become very high users of mental health services will benefit from assertive outreach and intensive input. Such services will be available seven days a week. It is intended to have 220 teams in place by 2004. **Assertive outreach services**

By December 2002, 191 Assertive Outreach teams had been developed.

By 2004, assertive outreach teams will be in place to provide support for everyone who needs it.

Encouraging progress has been made towards achieving the targets set for assertive outreach teams and establishing new workers and new ways of working. Progress towards establishing crisis resolution and early intervention teams is slower. Both crisis resolution and early intervention require a significant change in service culture in addition to reconfiguration.

Action taken since the last report includes

53. A Severe Mental Illness Project Team and its supporting Workgroups have continued to meet on a regular basis.

54. Service specifications for early intervention, crisis resolution and assertive outreach were issued as part of the Mental Health Policy Implementation Guide in March 2001. There is an ongoing process to seek to ensure that the NHS Plan commitments on these services are achieved.

55. Further guidance has been published in 2002. The first two items focused on good practice in acute in-patient care and outlined key recommendations within a ten-year plan, accompanied by national standards for psychiatric intensive care units. The third covered dual diagnosis services and provided a framework for all agencies involved in supporting people with mental health problems and substance misuse. A fourth document outlined a model service specification for Community Mental Health Teams.

56. All individuals who provide regular and substantial care for a person on CPA should: **…for carers**

- have an assessment of their caring, physical and mental health needs, repeated on at least an annual basis; **NSF standard six**

- have their own written care plan which is given to them and implemented in discussion with them.

Action taken since the last report includes

57. When carers are asked, what the majority want most is for mental health services to be provided around the clock. They also require time off from caring. This can reduce the social isolation that goes with the job – especially caring for someone with severe mental illness.

New staff will increase the breaks available for carers, and strengthen their support networks.

58. By October 2004, mental health services are expected to have identified and assessed all carers of those people with mental health problems as well as agreeing and implementing their carer support plans. It is also a NHS Plan commitment to recruit 700 more staff to increase the breaks available for carers and to strengthen carer support networks by 2004. To ensure that these targets are met, the Department has produced a leaflet 'A Commitment to Carers' that outlines the above position. In addition to this, the Department has developed guidelines on a service specification for support of carers of people with mental health problems.

By December 2002, guidance had been issued on carer support staff.

59. This specification is aimed at statutory and voluntary sector organisations who commission and provide services to people with mental health problems and their carers and families and its scope will include services to all carers of those people with mental health problems. It will be included in the Mental Health Policy Implementation Guide.

...for people at risk of self harm or suicide

NSF standard seven

60. Local health and social care communities should prevent suicides by:

- promoting mental health for all, working with individuals and communities (Standard one);

- delivering high quality primary mental health care (Standard two);

- ensuring that anyone with a mental health problem can contact local services via the primary care team, a helpline or an A&E department (Standard three);

- ensuring that individuals with severe and enduring mental illness have a care plan which meets their specific needs, including access to services round the clock (Standard four);

- providing safe hospital accommodation for individuals who need it (Standard five);

- enabling individuals caring for someone with severe mental illness to receive the support which they need to continue to care (Standard six).

and in addition:

- support local prison staff in preventing suicides among prisoners;

- ensure that staff are competent to assess the risk of suicide among individuals at greatest risk;

- develop local systems for suicide audit to learn lessons and take any necessary action.

61. Preventing suicide, or deliberate self-harm, is not an easy matter – but the Government has set a firm target to reduce the number of suicides by one fifth by 2010. The thrust of new mental health policy, and other Government policy, is to make society a better place to live, and to ensure that when people have mental health problems, there are safe, sound, supportive services available.

62. The first national suicide prevention strategy for England was launched on the 16 September 2002 to ensure that all is being done to prevent suicide in pursuit of the OHN target. The strategy was developed, under the direction of the National Director for Mental Health, Professor Louis Appleby, and followed publication of a consultation document in April 2002. Over 300 comments were received during the three-month consultation period which have helped to develop the strategy.

64. The strategy is a co-ordinated set of activities that will take place over several years, and it will evolve as new priorities and new evidence on prevention emerge. The strategy is intended to provide a coherent approach to suicide prevention, based on four key principles. It aims to be:

- Comprehensive

The strategy recognises that suicide prevention is not the exclusive responsibility of any one sector of society, or of health services alone. This is particularly important in mental health services. People with mental illness are at high risk and mental health services have a vital part to play; however, many people who commit suicide are not in contact with mental health services.

- Based on evidence

The strategy is intended to be evidence-based. It draws on published research wherever possible. Where the evidence is weak, it proposes to improve it.

- Specific

The strategy will be built around a number of actions. These are intended to be specific, practical and open to monitoring.

- Subject to evaluation

The strategy itself must be subject to continual evaluation and changed when necessary.

The document sets out as concisely as possible a proposal for a suicide prevention strategy for England, formulated by an expert advisory group through consultation with mental health professionals, researchers, survivors of suicide attempts, the voluntary sector and others with relevant experience. It follows a 3-month public consultation exercise. It sets out a programme of activity to reduce suicide based on six goals:

1. To reduce risk among key high-risk groups.

2. To promote mental well-being in the wider population.

3. To reduce the availability and lethality of suicidal methods.

4. To improve the reporting of suicidal behaviour in the media.

5. To promote research on suicide prevention.

6. To improve the monitoring of progress towards the *Saving Lives: Our Healthier Nation* target for reducing suicide.

Under each goal, a series of more precise objectives is proposed. For each of these, it describes:

- key actions already taken; and

- new actions to be taken.

64. In addition a range of other action has been taken including:

- reducing the pack sizes of paracetamol and aspirin;

- supporting people who are at high risk of suicide.

Since March 2002 all patients with a history of severe mental illness or deliberate self-harm, must be followed up, by personal contact with a mental health professional, within 7 days of discharge from hospital.

Since March 2002 psychiatric in-patient units must review their physical environment and reduce access to means of suicide.

65. The Department of Health, through the National Institute for Clinical Excellence, funds the National Confidential Inquiry into Suicide and Homicide by People with Mental Illness to ensure that everyone involved in mental health services learns and implements lessons from the factors associated with serious incidents. The Inquiry is crucial to gaining a better understanding of the circumstances surrounding homicides and suicides committed by people with mental illness. The Inquiry team published *Safety First: Five-Year Report of the National Confidential Inquiry into Suicide and Homicide by People with Mental Illness* in March 2001. The Department of Health is committed to taking appropriate action in response to the findings of the Inquiry.

66. The Department of Health has required services to reduce to zero by the end of March 2002 the number of suicides on acute psychiatric wards by ensuring that immediate action is taken to remove all non-collapsible structures such as bed, shower and curtain rails in all psychiatric in-patient settings. This has been achieved.

67. Focusing on high-risk groups, such as young men, is part of the Government's action to reduce the overall suicide rate. In December 1997 the Department of Health launched the CALM (Campaign Against Living Miserably) telephone helpline in Manchester. It provides a safety net for young men by breaking down the barriers and reducing the stigma attached to depression and mental illness. The helpline, aimed at young men between the ages of 15-35 offers advice, guidance, information and counselling at the onset of depression. The helpline has since been rolled out to Merseyside and Cumbria in March 2000, and Bedfordshire in May 2001, and we are looking to make it available in other areas in partnership with local agencies and authorities.

68. The Department of Health's *mind out for mental health* campaign, launched in March 2001, is a national anti-discrimination campaign designed to raise awareness of mental health issues and cut through the stigma and isolation which can so often lead to people taking their own lives.

By December 2002, suicide rates, whilst fluctuating year on year, show a downward trend since the early 1980s. The 2000 death rate was similar to the 1997 death rate, so the period 1998-2000 has a similar death rate to the period 1997-1999 (most recent data – using a 3-year rolling average).

DEVELOPMENT WORK FOR SPECIFIC CLIENT GROUPS

69. More women than men use mental health services, but services are not always sensitive to the specific needs of women. Women are more likely to suffer from anxiety, depression and eating disorders. One in ten have post-natal depression after childbirth. Women can be vulnerable when receiving care in a mixed sex environment. More attention is needed to the links between childhood sexual abuse and adult mental distress, particularly in women. Very few services are available at present for women who self harm.

For women

70. Too many women are kept in conditions of high security simply because no other service is available for them. The development of alternative services for patients who should not be detained in high secure hospitals is therefore of particular importance for women.

Strategic Health Authorities are expected to provide women-only community based day services – as well as providing women-only accommodation in hospital facilities.

Action taken since last report

71. The development of a women's strategy forms part of the Government's commitment to address inequalities in the delivery of mental health services. The aim of the consultation document *Women's Mental Health: Into the Mainstream* is to provide information, to generate discussion and to outline a strategic direction to mainstream women's mental health care needs. The public consultation, October to December 2002, provided an opportunity for the Department of Health to listen to the views of all stakeholders across health and social care. Written comments were invited and a number of listening events were held around the country. The document can be found at www.doh.gov.uk/mentalhealth/women.htm. Copies of the full-length version and/or summary can be obtained from: Department of Health, P.O. Box 777, London SE1 6XH, tel. 08701 555455, e-mail doh@prolog.uk.com

By December 2002, the strategy on improving services for women had been published and consulted on, including guidance for local services on women only day services.

72. For far too long, the needs of people from minority communities have not been adequately met by mainstream mental health services. The National Service Framework for Mental Health has identified this.

For people from minority ethnic groups

73. Many of the services outlined in the *NHS Plan* have proved to be accessible, and far more acceptable, to black and minority ethnic service users. However, services require further improvement.

Action taken since the last report

74. The Mental Health Task Force was asked to prepare recommendations on improving mental health services for black and minority ethnic groups. A report 'Inside/Outside; Improving Mental Health Services for Black and Minority Ethnic Communities in England' will was published in March 2003. An implementation framework to improve services in the area of ethnicity and mental health is being developed to take forward the work of 'Inside/Outside'.

In Improvement, Expansion and Reform: The Next 3 years Priorities and Planning Framework 2003 - 2006 (issued September 2002) a target had been set for placement of 500 Community Development Workers for Black and Minority Ethnic Communities.

For people in high security hospitals

Movement of inappropriately placed patients

75. The exercise to facilitate the movement of inappropriately placed patients out of the high security hospitals continues. This "accelerated discharge" programme, supported by additional capital and revenue funding, is aimed at moving up to 400 inappropriately placed patients from the high security hospitals to more suitable accommodation by 2004. Regional targets have been set for the numbers of patients to move and the movement process has begun. As part of this process, two hundred long-term secure beds are being developed to allow patients to move on. The aim is to move towards a situation in which the hospitals fulfil their true purpose of providing a service for people who require high security care at the time when they genuinely need it, with admission and discharge delays minimised.

Review of Security at the high security hospitals

76. Most of the recommendations of the Security Review Report have now been implemented. The main outstanding issues relate to the upgrading of the perimeter security of the hospitals, on which work is ongoing. The Report, compiled by a Team led by Sir Richard Tilt, the former Director General of the Prison Service, was published in May 2000. The Review covered all three high security hospitals and 86 recommendations were made, all of which were accepted by the Government. Implementation of the Report's recommendations is further improving the security of the high security hospitals for the benefit of the general public, staff and patients.

Integration of the high security hospitals into NHS Trusts

77. All three high security hospitals have integrated into NHS Trusts during the past couple of years. Broadmoor Hospital became part of the West London Mental Health NHS Trust with effect from 1 April 2001, and Rampton Hospital became part of the Nottinghamshire Healthcare NHS Trust from the same date. Ashworth Hospital became part of the Mersey Care NHS Trust with effect from 1 April 2002. Performance management of the hospitals is now undertaken by Strategic Health Authorities (StHAs) (Cheshire and Merseyside for Ashworth Hospital, North West London for Broadmoor Hospital and Trent for Rampton Hospital).

Arrangements for the commissioning and performance management of high security psychiatric services

78. The arrangements for the commissioning and performance management of high security psychiatric services have been reviewed in the light of the wider changes taking place in the NHS as a result of the Shifting the Balance of Power process. For 2002-03, the existing arrangements whereby high and medium secure psychiatric services are commissioned through the Regional Specialised Commissioning arrangements is continuing but the High Security Psychiatric Services Commissioning National Oversight Group, which ensures that the Secretary of State's duty under Section 4 of the NHS Act 1977 to provide high security psychiatric services is properly discharged, has been streamlined and revised Cluster and Catchment Group arrangements introduced. The commissioning arrangements will be revisited when the current review of the process for commissioning specialised services more widely is completed.

Review of the Child Visiting Directions

79. The high security hospital Child Visiting Directions were introduced in July 1999 in the light of the findings of the Committee of Inquiry into the Personality Disorder Unit at

Ashworth Hospital. Selected aspects of these Directions and their subsequent amendments were the subject of a consultation exercise, which ended on 6 September 2002. The consultation responses are in the process of being considered, with a view to considering what changes are required to the existing Directions.

Arrangements for social work provision in the high security hospitals

80. During the past year considerable progress has been made in implementing the recommendations of the Lewis Report, *Review of Social Work Service in the High Security Hospitals*. Arrangements have been made in the case of Broadmoor and Rampton Hospitals for the social work service to be managed by local authorities. Discussions about the arrangements to be made in respect of Ashworth Hospital are ongoing. The Department of Health, working with representatives of a wide range of interests, developed a set of *National Standards for the provision of Social Care Services in the High Security Hospitals* (August 2001). This was published with a covering letter by the Chief Inspector of Social Services, which identified 20 key standards to be implemented by 31 March 2003.

For people in prison

81. At any time about 5,000 people with a serious mental illness are in prison. It is important to improve the detection and treatment of prisoners' mental health problems. New partnerships, between the NHS and local prisons, will employ some 300 additional staff.

All people in prison who have severe mental illness will receive treatment, and none will leave prison without a care plan and a care co-ordinator.

Action taken since the last report

82. The Prison Mental Health Strategy was published in December 2001. Changing the Outlook; A Strategy for Developing and Modernising Mental Health Services in Prison outlines where mental health services in prison are expected to be in the next 3 to 5 years, and emphasises that change can only be achieved if the Prison Service and Department of Health work together in partnership.

83. The prison mental health in-reach project, established to implement commitments made in the NHS Plan, is now in its second financial year. 22 prisons in England and Wales have joined the project during 2001/02. Of these 22 prisons, 4 are in Wales, and the remainder are made up of a combination of Local prisons, Women's prisons, Young Offender Institutes and High Secure establishments. A further 25 establishments are to come on stream in the current financial year to produce a total of 47 by the end of 2002/3. The plan is to extend the in-reach project to include around 70 prisons who are judged to have the greatest mental health need by 2004, which should encompass the estimated 5,000 people in the prison system at any one time with severe and enduring mental illness. The in-reach teams provide similar services to those that Community Mental Health Teams provide in the community.

In Improvement, Expansion and Reform: The Next 3 years Priorities and Planning Framework 2003 - 2006 (issued September 2002) a target had been set of employing 300 prison in-reach staff by 2004. By December 2002, 150 prison in-reach staff had been employed. A target for an additional 300 staff has also been set for 2006.

84. As part of the in-reach project, the Mental Health Expert Group was established in 2001 to oversee the project and provide multi-agency support and advice. The Expert Group is chaired by Professor Louis Appleby, the Government's National Director for Mental Health, and has members from the Department of Health, the Prison Service, the Youth

Justice Board, NACRO, the Home Office, Royal College of Psychiatry and the National Assembly for Wales, as well as practitioners working in the prison mental health field.

85. In November 2002, the Prison Mental Health Expert Group launched a Prison Mental Health Collaborative. The Collaborative is an established approach, which is used to empower staff to modernise clinical services. Primarily the Collaborative will set up a structure in which good practice will be shared and provide peer support. The Collaborative aims to identify training needs and empower staff to make decisions about their service.

For people with severe personality disorder

86. A very small number of people, who have a severe personality disorder, pose a risk to other patients, staff, and the public as well as to themselves. Suitable services have not been available to help such people, or to manage their behaviour. The role of the current Mental Health Act is not clear, either.

87. Specialist help for this group of people is being developed, in local mental health services, in regional forensic services, in high secure hospitals and in prisons. A programme of research and evaluation is backing this up. New legislation will set out clearer powers to manage people who pose a serious risk of significant harm to others as a result of their mental disorder, including those with severe personality disorder.

88. The aim is to help individuals – many of whom are also among the most needy and disadvantaged people in our society – to accept responsibility for their problems and, by changing their behaviour, work towards successful re-integration into the community.

By 2004, an additional 140 places in high secure hospitals together with provision in medium secure units and community hostels will be provided for people with severe personality disorder. By December 2002, work on meeting this target was in progress.

Action taken since the last report

- Progress has been made in planning the development of new units for the assessment and treatment of people who are dangerous and have severe personality disorder at Broadmoor and Rampton. These will open in 2004, and provide 140 places.

- A range of pilot provision is being created in medium secure and community settings, including medium secure beds, community teams and community hostel places, sited in the North East and in London. This provision will come on stream in 2004.

- A strategy for Personality Disorder was issued in January 2003 (http://www.doh.gov.uk/mentalhealth/personalitydisorder.htm), and provides the blueprint for the future development of services.

For Child and Adolescent mental health services

The children's NSF

89. In February 2001 the Secretary of State for Health announced the intention to produce a Children's National Service Framework (NSF) to develop new national standards across the NHS and social services for children (including maternity services). It was subsequently confirmed that the NSF would have a significant component covering child and adolescent mental health services (CAMHS). The new standards will help to ensure that children and young people are able to access appropriate services at the right time and that they can take an active part in making decisions about their care. The work will be led by Professor Al Aynsley-Green, chairman of the Children's Taskforce and National Clinical Director for Children. The Children's Taskforce is overseeing the development of the NSF.

90. As a result of targeted funding (£105 million over 3 years to March 2003) given to support the CAMHS development strategy, including grants to twenty four innovative local projects, there has been increased provision, e.g. in terms of more staff and new or enhanced services, and good service models are emerging. However, service pressures are increasing as are the expectations of other agencies and programmes. The CAMHS module of the Children's NSF will be the main focus in taking forward the future stages of CAMHS development.

91. The Department of Health's new mental health Public Service Agreement (PSA) target sets an agenda to improve significantly the services for children and young people with mental health problems. The target is to:

New CAMHS targets

- improve life outcomes of adults and children with mental health problems through year on year improvements in access to crisis and CAMHS services, and reduce the mortality rate from suicide and undetermined injury by at least 20% by 2010.

92. The expectations and capacity assumptions underpinning this target are:

- The Children's National Service Framework and its emerging findings will set out the standards and milestones for improvement in CAMHS services, including year on year improvements in access.

- All CAMHS to provide a comprehensive service including mental health promotion and early intervention by 2006.

- Increase CAMHS by at least 10 per cent each year across the service according to agreed local priorities. (Demonstrated by increased staffing, patient contacts and/or investment.)

Older people with Mental Health Problems

93. The National Service Framework (NSF) for older people was published on 27 March 2001 and sets out new national standards of care for older people, including those with mental health problems.

For Older people with a mental health problem - the Older Persons National Service Framework Standard 7

94. Standard seven of the NSF is devoted to requirements relating to the mental health needs of older people - and this focuses on dementia and depression. The standard sets out what types of services should be provided for people with dementia and their carers by the NHS and councils - access to integrated mental health services to ensure effective diagnosis, treatment and support

95. By April 2004, Primary Care Trusts will have ensured that every general practice uses protocols agreed with local specialist services, both health and social care, to diagnose, treat and care for patients with depression or dementia. Health and social care systems should have agreed protocols in place for the care and management of older people with mental health problems

96. Mental health problems are common among older people. At any one time, around 10-15% of the population aged 65 and over has depression. About 5% of people aged 65 and over have dementia. Among people aged 80 and above, this rises to 20%.

97. Work is underway to implement the NSF and in particular standard 7. Support is provided centrally in a number of ways, for example:

(i) the Department is providing Section 64 funding to the voluntary sector to support a range of projects to develop dementia services;

(ii) the Government provides support for a range of different research projects relating to the mental health needs of older people;

(iii) work is being carried out to see what needs to be done to develop – in terms of numbers and skills - the workforce to enable the field to implement the NSF. Work is also taking place on piloting new ways of working in dementia services, to ensure that the best use is made of the resources available and that services are delivered in a person-centred, integrated way;

(iv) a new Single Assessment Process for older people has been published; and

(v) we are working closely with the range of different organisations with an interest in standard 7.

We will be monitoring against the milestones in the NSF to ensure that progress is made as required.

For people who are mentally ill and experience hearing problems

98. The Department of Health launched a consultation document, "A Sign of the Times" in July 2002 that set out a number of recommendations and options for improving services for Deaf people with mental health problems.

99. The document covers all age groups and considers how this disadvantaged group could receive the same level of preventative, primary, secondary and specialist provision as the hearing population.

100. The consultation ended in October 2002.

For people who are admitted to acute in-patient settings

101. Jacqui Smith MP, Minister of State for Health, launched the Department's guidance on Acute Inpatient Care, which has been produced following careful consideration of existing evidence and good practice, as well as through extensive consultation with clinicians, managers and other organisations involved in Mental Health. It outlines key recommendations and standards of care within a ten year plan which include standards for psychiatric intensive care units.

102. The specific education and training implications are being reviewed, and will be progressed to provide a supporting framework for practitioner development, contributing to improved services and quality of care for those who require an episode of in patient admission.

OTHER SUPPORTING DEVELOPMENTS

For the voluntary sector

Financial Support to the Mental Illness Voluntary Sector

103. Under Section 64 of the Health Services and Public Health Act 1968, the Department of Health awards grants towards the administrative costs of national voluntary organisations as well as supporting national development projects or innovative local projects with potential for national replication. For 2002/03, 99 grants were awarded to 63 voluntary organisations in respect of adult and elderly mental health at a total cost of nearly £3.5 million. In addition, organisations providing Child and Adolescent Mental Health services were awarded grants amounting to over £340,000 to fund projects and core services.

104. The grants currently payable to the voluntary sector provide a broad package of support. For example, they cover a number of client groups such as older people, women, mentally disordered offenders and black and minority ethnic people as well as users; they are spread amongst organisations both large and small and they cover a number of different forms of mental illness including (manic) depression, schizophrenia, phobias, effects of trauma and eating disorders. In addition, they support a number of key Government and Departmental policies and priorities such as the New Deal initiative, prevention of suicide, working across organisational boundaries and tackling social exclusion.

Mental Health Beacons **Beacons**

105. As part of the Modernisation Agency, the NHS Beacon Programme supports the development of a modern, responsive health service where patients have access to faster, more convenient and more appropriate care. By identifying services that have been particularly innovative in meeting specific health care needs and encouraging them to share their experience via a flexible Beacon Programme, others can benefit by using or adapting original ideas to suit their own circumstances, saving time and resources and avoiding duplication of effort. Each Beacon receives money to help promoting the programme of a wide range of learning opportunities to match team and individual needs, including workshops, conferences, visits, mentoring and secondments. All current Beacons are showcased on the Programme website at www.nhs.uk/beacons.

106. In the area of mental health, the NHS Beacon Programme has to date identified 49 examples of good practice. Many of these were nominated for Nye Bevan awards (now known as Health and Social Care Awards) designed to recognise and celebrate teams who have modernised their services. In 1999, 35 were chosen in mental health including 8 Nye Bevan awards as being amongst the very best beacons. Two mental health services were among the Nye award winners: North Birmingham Mental Health Trust and the community mental health service in North Kirklees. North Kirklees won the prize for best beacon service overall.

107. A further 14 Beacon sites were chosen in mental health in 2000. In the Nye Bevan Awards for 2000, the winner of the Northern and Yorkshire Regional Modernisation Award (and runner up for the National award) was the OPUS Employment project run by Northumberland Mental Health Trust. Another Beacon, Barrow Community Gym (led by Bay Community NHS Trust) was the runner-up in the same category in the North-West Region.

108. The funding for Mental Health Beacons successful in 1999 ended in 2001. Owing to the success of the 1999 Beacons (the first tranche for mental health) they were invited to apply for an extension of funding in 2001/02. 19 were successful and received funds to continue their programme into 2001/02. No further Mental Health Beacons have come on stream in 2002/03.

109. Following an evaluation of the success of the Beacon programme the Modernisation Agency is now looking to conduct a national pilot with a new approach to Beacons. This should come on stream later this year.

110. NHS Direct has made significant progress in addressing the needs of callers with **NHS Direct** mental health concerns. Over 800 nurse advisors have been trained to assess the needs of callers and this includes as assessment of risk of self-harm. Every NHS Direct call centre has a lead mental health nurse, two have experienced mental health social workers. All nurse advisors are able to access support and clinical supervision on site. Training on mental health is now part of the induction programme for all new staff and on-going up date

training is also provided on a regular basis. Protocols for referral in a crisis have been established with the majority of mental health providers. Work is progressing to establish a protocol for the exchange of information between NHS Direct and Trusts to enable NHS Direct to support on-going care for service users on enhanced CPA. A review of mental health algorithms has been completed and additional mental health algorithms are being developed in collaboration with clinical colleagues.

Inquiries

111. The Health Service Guidance released in 1994 creates a requirement for a formal inquiry after any homicide by a person with a mental illness. Since 1994, with changing services and changing public expectations this guidance has been found in need of updating. Families of victims of homicide have not felt involved and part of the process, staff have felt victimised by it, and it has proved unsuccessful in supporting and enabling the organisational changes which are needed to stop such incidents happening again.

In the light of this the Guidance is begin reviewed, with key stakeholders, with a review to replacing the guidance in 2003.

Work with other Government Departments

112. The mental health branch of the Department of Health has been working to ensure that mental health areas are being picked up within the National Institute for Clinical Excellence (NICE) work programme. The following guidelines are under development: 1) Management of schizophrenia; 2) Management of depression; 3) Management of eating disorders; 4) Anxiety: management of generalised anxiety disorder and panic disorder (with or without agoraphobia) in adults in primary, secondary and community care; 5) Disturbed (violent) behaviour: the short-term management of disturbed (violent) behaviour in inpatient psychiatric settings; 6) Management of self-harm. Appraisals are underway of the clinical and cost effectiveness of 1) the use of Computerised Cognitive Behaviour Therapy in anxiety and depression; 2) the use of ECT in depression, schizophrenia, catatonia and mania; 3) the use of new drugs in bipolar disorder; 4) the use of atypical antipsychotics in schizophrenia. An appraisal has been published on the use of Donepezil, Rivastigmine and Galantamine in Alzheimer's disease and the use of methylphenidate in Attention Deficit Hyperactivity Disorder in those under 16 years of age.

World Mental Health Day

113. World Mental Health Day (WMHD) is celebrated all over the world on 10 October each year. It provides a unique opportunity for a wide variety of groups and organisations to raise awareness about mental health. For WMHD 2001 and 2002, the Department of Health supported the network of local organisers engaged in promoting mental health through the *mind out for mental health* campaign. A local activist pack with ideas for practical action on and beyond WMHD was made available. It included facts about mental health and advice on how to arrange local events and secure local media coverage. It also included a listing of all the free materials available, including posters, leaflets and the campaign tag.

MAKING IT HAPPEN

114. The *NHS Plan* and the *National Service Framework* have set out some radical changes to mental health care. To make sure these changes happen – and that the people who use services feel the difference – will take a lot of effort, over several years, with everybody concerned working well together.

Planning change together

115. At national level the changes are being overseen by a new Mental Health Taskforce Board. It includes representatives of Government, the NHS and social services, service users and voluntary groups.

116. Professor Louis Appleby is the National Director for Mental Health, and chairs the Task Force. Senior staff at the Department of Health are co-ordinating national work for each NSF standard, as well as for the essential "underpinning programmes" of workforce, information, and research and development.

117. The Mental Health Task Force aims to develop mental health services that are planned and delivered around the needs and aspirations of service users, and specifically that: **Mental Health Task Force Mission Statement**

- treat individuals living with mental health problems with dignity and encourage their full involvement in their care;

- respect cultural and ethnic diversity and tackle discriminatory practices;

- respect the role and skills of carers, acknowledging them as partners in care and supporting them in this role;

- promote positive mental health and take effective steps to reduce stigma and discrimination;

- make the best and most effective treatments available, when and where they are needed;

- respond appropriately to need, so that people with acute illness receive prompt access to care, and so that those with a broad range of health and social needs – including housing, occupation and finance – receive comprehensive care;

- emphasise safety, particularly of service users themselves; and

- are delivered by a workforce who are skilled, of high morale and able to adopt new ways of working.

118. NIMHE is the key vehicle that supports implementation of national mental health policy in England. It works with all agencies and interests to develop a co-ordinated programme of research, service development, workforce development and support. NIMHE is part of the Modernisation Agency and takes the lead within the agency for programmes on mental health. NIMHE places the needs of service users, families and carers at the heart of its practice. **National Institute for Mental Health in England (NIMHE)**

119. NIMHE has four elements:

1. a small administrative centre which oversees and support the work of NIMHE;

2. Development Centres: NIMHE has established eight development centres in different parts of the country, which will be the main contact point for local practitioners. The regional centres will work along a wide network of local stakeholders and providing practical support to service development. Some of these centres have grown out of existing mental health organisations and some are new.

3. a National Mental Health Research Network; and

4. a series of time-limited programmes, for example to further develop mental health services in primary care.

120. NIMHE is led by the Chief Executive (Professor Antony Sheehan).

121. The first wave of work to be carried out by NIMHE was announced on World Mental Health Day 2002 and includes:

- the establishment of a mental health research network (MHRN) as a standing programme of NIMHE;

- within the research responsibilities of NIMHE two research projects will be initiated, a trail of assertive outreach in the UK and an examination of workload issues for mental health professionals;

- the commissioning of work to draw together existing good practice in service user evaluation and publish a kit of tools and systems for service user focused monitoring;

- in collaboration with the Sainsbury Centre for Mental Health Training a National Training & Development Programme for Assertive Outreach & Crisis Resolution Teams will be put in place;

- the production of a mental health promotion toolkit for primary care; and

- The development of a national consensus on values for mental health.

122. NIMHE will also be setting up a series of core programmes – acute inpatient care, community teams, equalities, intelligence in progress, primary care, research network, substance misuse, suicide prevention and workforce.

123. In partnership with other mental health organisations, NIMHE will be appointing Fellowships for expert advice. Fellows will be appointed in social care, young people, older people, experts by experience and recovery, Fellows are intended to encourage a national profile and partnership with relevant organisations; and the development of both research and good practice.

124. More can be found out about NIMHE at http://www.nimhe.org.uk/priorities.asp

Policy Implementation Guide

125. The Implementation Guide for adult mental health services was launched in March 2001. It included evidence based information and guidance to support local services develop new community mental health services, such as assertive outreach, home treatment and early intervention teams.

Since then, further guidance was published in 2002 covering:

- Adult acute inpatient care provision;

- National minimum standards for psychiatric intensive care units and low secure environments;

- Dual diagnosis good practice guidance;

- Community Mental Health Teams;

- Developing services for carers.

126. At local level, in each health and social care community, there is a local implementation team (LIT) to plan and deliver change. It too comprises the statutory services (such as health, social services and housing) for the area, together with service users, carers, and local voluntary groups that either provide care themselves, or campaign for better mental health care.

Local Implementation Teams

Published by TSO (The Stationery Office) and available from:

Online
www.tso.co.uk/bookshop

Mail, Telephone, Fax & E-mail
TSO
PO Box 29, Norwich NR3 1GN
Telephone orders/General enquiries 0870 600 5522
Fax orders 0870 600 5533
Order through the Parliamentary Hotline Lo-call 0845 7 023474
E-mail book.orders@tso.co.uk
Textphone 0870 240 3701

TSO Shops
123 Kingsway, London WC2B 6PQ
020 7242 6393 Fax 020 7242 6394
68-69 Bull Street, Birmingham B4 6AD
0121 236 9696 Fax 0121 236 9699
9-21 Princess Street, Manchester M60 8AS
0161 834 7201 Fax 0161 833 0634
16 Arthur Street, Belfast BT1 4GD
028 9023 8451 Fax 028 9023 5401
18-19 High Street, Cardiff CF10 1PT
029 2039 5548 Fax 029 2038 4347
71 Lothian Road, Edinburgh EH3 9AZ
0870 606 5566 Fax 0870 606 5588

The Parliamentary Bookshop
12 Bridge Street, Parliament Square,
London SW1A 2JX
Telephone orders/General enquiries 020 7219 3890
Fax orders 020 7219 3866

TSO Accredited Agents
(see Yellow Pages)

and through good booksellers

ISBN 0-10-292273-X